I0490846

The Unlocked Secret of Weight Loss

The Future of Obesity Treatment

By
Dr. Joanna Wells

Book review

" The Unlocked Secret of Weight Loss" by Dr. Joanna Wells is a comprehensive guide to losing weight and maintaining a healthy lifestyle. The book is designed to help readers understand the science behind weight loss, the psychological factors that contribute to weight gain and the practical strategies that can be used to achieve lasting weight loss.

One of the key strengths of the book is its emphasis on the psychological aspects of weight loss. The author recognizes that many people struggle with emotional eating and other psychological barriers to weight loss, and she provides practical advice and strategies for overcoming these challenges.

The book also includes a number of helpful tools and resources, including a food plan, recipes, and a variety of exercises and activities.

Another strength of the book is its focus on sustainable weight loss. The author emphasizes the importance of making gradual lifestyle changes rather than relying on quick-fix diets or extreme measures. By emphasizing the importance of long-term sustainability, the book provides readers with a roadmap for achieving and maintaining a healthy weight over the long term.

Overall, "The unlocked Secret of Weight Loss" is a well-written and informative book that provides readers with a comprehensive guide to weight loss and healthy living. Whether you are just starting out on your weight loss journey or looking for new strategies to maintain your weight loss, this book is an excellent resource that is sure to provide you with the tools and guidance you need to achieve your goals.

Disclaimer

The information contained in "The unlocked Secret of Weight Loss" by Joanna Wells is for educational purposes only and is not intended as a substitute for professional medical advice, diagnosis, or treatment. Always seek the advice of your physician or other qualified healthcare providers with any questions you may have regarding a medical condition or before embarking on a weight loss program.

The author and publisher of this book make no representations or warranties with respect to the accuracy, applicability, fitness, or completeness of the contents of this book.

Joanna Wells is the sole proprietor of the book.

The information in this book is based on research and personal experience, but the effectiveness of any weight loss program will vary depending on individual circumstances and adherence to the program.

The reader should consult with a healthcare professional before starting any weight loss program or making any significant changes to their diet or exercise routine.

Table of content

2.
1.
2.
3.

-
  A.
  B.
  C.
  D.

-
  A.
  B.
  C.
  D.

-
  A.
  B.
  C.

-
  A.
  B.
  C.
  D.

-
  A.
  B
  C.
  D.

-
  A.
  B.
  C.

  A.
  B.

Introduction

1. Definition of weight loss;

Weight loss refers to the reduction in body weight resulting from a loss of body fat, muscle mass, or both. It can occur intentionally through changes in diet and physical activity or unintentionally due to an underlying medical condition. The amount of weight loss varies depending on the individual's starting weight, lifestyle habits, and the methods used to achieve the weight loss. A healthy rate of obesity loss is generally considered to be 1-2 pounds per week. Weight loss can have numerous benefits for overall health, such as improving cardiovascular health, reducing the risk of chronic diseases, and improving mental well-being. However, extreme or rapid weight loss can also be harmful and should be avoided.

B. Benefits of weight loss

Weight loss can be important for so many kinds of reasons, including:

1. Improved overall health: Losing weight can reduce the risk of a number of health conditions, including heart disease, diabetes, high blood pressure, and certain types of cancer. It can also improve sleep, mobility, and overall quality of life.

2. Increased energy: Carrying excess weight can make you feel sluggish and tired. Losing weight can help increase your energy levels, making it easier to stay active and engaged in daily activities.

3. Improved mental health: Losing weight can improve self-esteem and confidence, which can have a positive impact on mental health. It can also reduce symptoms of depression and anxiety.

4. Increased lifespan: Maintaining a healthy weight can increase your lifespan, as obesity

has been linked to a shorter life expectancy.

5. Improved fertility: Obesity can have a negative impact on fertility in both men and women. Losing weight can improve fertility and increase the chances of conceiving.

6. Reduced healthcare costs: Obesity and its associated health conditions can be expensive to treat. Losing weight can reduce healthcare costs and improve long-term health outcomes.

Overall, weight loss can have numerous benefits for both physical and mental health, making it an important goal for many individuals. However, it is important to approach weight loss in a healthy and sustainable way, with a focus on long-term lifestyle changes rather than quick fixes or fad diets.

C. Weight loss principles

The basic principles of weight loss involve creating a caloric deficit, increasing physical activity, and making healthy food choices. Here are some more detailed explanations of these principles:

1. Caloric deficiency: To lose weight, you need to burn more calories than you consume. This can be obtained only by reducing the intake of calories, increasing your physical activity, or a combination of both. A safe and sustainable rate of weight loss is generally 1-2 pounds per week, which equates to a caloric deficit of 500-1000 calories per day.

2. Physical activity: Regular exercise can help you burn more calories, increase muscle mass, and improve your overall health. Aim for at least 150 minutes of moderate-intensity aerobic exercise per week, such as brisk walking or cycling, along with strength-training exercises at least twice per week.

3. Healthy food choices: Choosing nutrient-dense foods that are low in calories can help you feel full and satisfied while reducing your overall calorie intake. Focus on eating plenty of fruits, vegetables, lean proteins, and whole grains, and limit your intake of processed foods, sugary drinks, and high-fat foods.

Other factors that can affect weight loss include genetics, hormones, sleep, stress, and medication use. It's important to work with a healthcare provider or registered dietitian to develop a personalized weight loss plan that takes these factors into account and is safe and effective for you.

Chapter 1

Understanding calories

A.What are calories

Calories are a measure of energy. Specifically, a calorie is a unit of energy that is commonly used to describe the amount of energy provided by food and drink. The calorie is defined as the amount of energy required to raise the temperature of one gram of water by one degree Celsius.

When we talk about calories in the context of nutrition, we are usually referring to kilocalories, which are often abbreviated as "kcal" or simply calories. One kilocalorie is equal to 1,000 calories, so when we say that a food contains 100 calories, we really mean that it contains 0.1 kilocalories (or 1000 calories). When we eat food, our bodies use the energy from the calories in that food to power all of our daily activities, from breathing and circulating blood to exercising and thinking. The number of calories we need each day depends on a variety of factors, including our age, gender, height, weight, and activity level.

B.Calories in and out.

Calorie intake and expenditure are important concepts related to maintaining a healthy weight and overall health.

Calorie intake refers to the amount of energy (in the form of calories) that is consumed through food and drinks. This energy is used by the body to perform various functions, such as physical activity, maintaining body temperature, and supporting organ function.

Calorie expenditure refers to the amount of energy that is burned by the body through physical activity and basic bodily functions such as breathing and digestion. The amount of calorie expenditure can vary based on factors such as age, sex, weight, height, and level of physical activity.

 To maintain a healthy weight: it is important to balance calorie intake with calorie expenditure. If the amount of calories consumed is greater than the number of calories burned, this can lead to weight gain. On the other hand, if the amount of calories burned is greater than the number of calories consumed, this can lead to weight loss.

Therefore, it is important to have a healthy and balanced diet that provides the necessary nutrients and calories for the body, as well as engaging in regular physical activity to assist with burning calories and maintaining healthy fat.

C. How to calculate your daily calorie needs:

Calculating your daily calorie needs can be done using a few different methods, but one commonly used equation is the Harris-Benedict equation. This equation takes into account your age, sex, weight, and height to estimate your daily calorie needs. The Harris-Benedict equation is different for men and women, so use the appropriate formula based on your gender:

For men:

BMR = 88.36 + (13.4 x weight in kg) + (4.8 x height in cm) - (5.7 x age in years)

For women:

BMR = 447.6 + (9.2 x weight in kg) + (3.1 x height in cm) - (4.3 x age in years)

Once you have calculated your basal metabolic rate (BMR) using one of the above formulas, you can use an activity factor to estimate your daily calorie needs based on your level of physical activity:

Sedentary (little or no activity to perform): BMR x 1.2

Lightly active (exercise 1-3 days per week): BMR x 1.375

Effectively active (exercise 3-5 days a week): BMR x 1.55

Perfectly active (exercise 6-7 days a week): BMR x 1.725

Extra active (very hard exercise or physical activity): BMR x 1.9
For example, if you are a 30-year-old woman who weighs 65 kg, is 165 cm tall, and exercises moderately 3-5 days per week, your estimated daily calorie needs would be:

BMR = 447.6 + (9.2 x 65) + (3.1 x 165) - (4.3 x 30) = 1403.5 calories

Daily calorie needs = 1403.5 x 1.55 = 2174 calories

Remember that these calculations are only estimates and may not be accurate for everyone. It is important to listen to your body and adjust your calorie intake based on your individual needs and goals.

D.Understanding macronutrients and their calorie content:

Macronutrients are the essential nutrients required by the body in large amounts to perform various functions such as energy production, growth, and repair. The three macronutrients are carbohydrates, proteins, and fats, each of which has a different calorie content per gram.

1. Carbohydrates: Carbohydrates are the basic source of energy for the body. They are most likely to be found in foods like bread, pasta, rice, fruits, and vegetables. Carbohydrates provide a maximum of 4 calories per gram.

2. Proteins: Proteins are the building blocks of the body, necessary for growth and repair. They are found in foods like meat, fish, eggs, beans, and nuts. Proteins provide four calories per gram.

3. Fats: Fats are effectively necessary for the storage of energy and insulation. They are found in foods like butter, oil, nuts, and cheese. Fats provide nine calories per gram.

It's essential to consume a balanced diet containing all three macronutrients in the right proportions to meet your daily energy and nutritional needs. Consuming too much of any macronutrient, especially fats, and carbohydrates can lead to weight gain, while not consuming enough can lead to nutritional deficiencies and low energy levels.

Chapter 2

Nutrition and diet

A. The role of diet in weight loss
B. Understanding the food groups and their importance

Understanding the food groups is important for maintaining a balanced and healthy diet. There are five main food groups:

1. Fruits: Fruits are known for their wonderful source of vitamins, minerals, and fiber. They are low in fat and calories and can help to prevent chronic diseases such as heart disease and cancer. Fruits include apples, bananas, oranges, berries, melons, and many others.

2. Vegetables: Vegetables are an incredible part of a healthy and safeguarded diet. They are rich in vitamins, minerals, and fiber, and also can help to lower the risk of chronic diseases. Vegetables include leafy greens, carrots, peppers, broccoli, and many others.

3. Grains: Grains are an important source of carbohydrates, which provide energy for the body. Whole grains are especially beneficial, as they are high in fiber and can help to lower cholesterol and prevent heart disease. Grains include bread, pasta, rice, oats, and others.

4. Protein: Protein is essential for the building and repairing of body tissues. Good sources of protein include lean meats, poultry, fish, beans, nuts, and soy products.

5. Dairy: Dairy products are a good source of calcium, which is important for building and maintaining strong bones. Low-cholesterol dairy products such as milk, yogurt, and cheese are advisably prescribed.

It is important to eat a variety of foods from each of these food groups to ensure that your body is getting all of the nutrients it needs. Additionally, it is important to pay attention to portion sizes and limit the intake of processed and high-fat foods.

C. The importance of protein control

Protein is an essential macronutrient that is required by the body for a variety of functions, including building and repairing tissues, producing hormones and enzymes, and supporting immune function. Protein control refers to the management of protein intake to ensure that the body is receiving an adequate amount of protein without consuming excessive amounts. This is important for several reasons:

1. Muscle building and maintenance: Protein is necessary for the growth and maintenance of muscle tissue. If you are engaging in regular physical activity or trying to build muscle, consuming adequate amounts of protein is essential to support these goals.

2. Weight management: Protein can help to promote feelings of fullness and reduce appetite, which can help to support weight management goals. Additionally, a high-protein diet has been

shown to help preserve lean muscle mass during weight loss.

3. Healthy aging: As we age, our bodies become less efficient at utilizing protein. Adequate protein intake can help to support healthy aging by promoting muscle mass and strength, which can help to maintain mobility and independence.

4. Immune function: Protein is necessary for the production of antibodies and other immune system components, which help to protect the body against infection and disease.

It is important to note that excessive protein intake can be harmful to the body, particularly if it is coming from animal sources that are high in saturated fat. Additionally, those with certain health conditions, such as kidney disease, may need to limit their protein intake.

Therefore, it is important to work with a healthcare provider or registered dietitian to determine the appropriate level of protein intake for your individual needs.

D. Healthy Eating Strategies

Here are some strategies for healthier eating:

Plan your meals: Plan your meals for the week ahead of time. This will help you to avoid making unhealthy food choices when you are hungry and pressed for time.

1. Choose whole foods: Choose whole, unprocessed foods whenever possible. Whole foods are more nutritious and contain fewer additives and preservatives than processed foods.

2. Increase your intake of fruits and vegetables: Fruits and vegetables are rich in nutrients and fiber, and can help you to feel full and satisfied. Aim for at least five meals of fruits and vegetables in a day.

3. Limit your intake of sugary and high-fat foods: These foods can be high in calories and low in nutrients. Try to limit your intake of sugary and high-fat foods and choose healthier options instead.

4. Eat protein with every meal: Protein can help you to feel full and satisfied and can also help to build and repair muscles. Include protein-rich foods like lean meat,

fish, eggs, beans, and nuts in every meal.

5. Watch your portion sizes: Pay attention to portion sizes and try to eat smaller, more frequent meals throughout the day. This can help you to avoid overeating and can keep your metabolism running smoothly.

6. Stay hydrated: Drink plenty of water throughout the day to help keep your body hydrated and your digestion running smoothly.

7. Cook at home: Cooking at home can help you to control the ingredients and portion sizes of your meals, and can also save you money.

8. Be mindful of your eating habits: Pay attention to your hunger and fullness cues, and try to eat slowly and mindfully. This can help you to enjoy your food more and to avoid overeating.

9. Seek professional help if needed: If you are struggling to make healthy eating choices, consider seeking professional help from a registered dietitian or nutritionist. They can provide specialist advice and support in assisting you to reach your goals.

Chapter 3

Exercises and physical activity

Exercise can play an important role in weight loss by helping to burn calories and build muscle mass. When you engage in physical activity, you burn calories, and the more intense the exercise, the more calories you burn. This can create a calorie deficit, which means you burn more calories than you consume through your diet, leading to weight loss.

Exercise can also help to build muscle mass. The more muscle you have, the more calories you burn at rest, even when you're not exercising. This is because muscle tissue is metabolically active, meaning it requires energy to maintain.

In addition to burning calories and building muscle, exercise can also help to improve your overall health and well-being. Regular physical activity has been shown to reduce the risk of chronic diseases such as heart disease, diabetes, and certain types of cancer.

It's important to note, however, that exercise alone is not enough for weight loss. To achieve sustainable weight loss, it's essential to combine regular exercise with a healthy, balanced diet that provides the right amount of calories and nutrients for your body. Additionally, it's important to find an exercise routine that you enjoy and can stick to long-term, as consistency is key when it comes to weight loss and overall health.

B. Types of exercise needed for weight loss

When it comes to weight loss, it's important to focus on exercises that burn calories and increase your metabolic rate. Here are some types of exercise that can help with weight loss:

1. Cardiovascular exercise: Also known as cardio, this type of exercise involves activities that increase your heart rate and

breathing, such as running, cycling, swimming, or brisk walking. Cardio helps burn calories and can boost your metabolism.

High-Intensity Interval Training (HIIT): HIIT involves short bursts of intense exercise followed by periods of rest. This type of exercise can help you burn more calories in a shorter amount of time and can also increase your metabolic rate.

2. Strength Training: Building muscle can help increase your metabolic rate and burn more calories. Strength training exercises include weightlifting, bodyweight exercises, or using resistance bands.

3. Circuit Training: This type of workout combines strength training and cardio exercises to create a full-body workout that can help you burn calories and build muscle.

4. Yoga or Pilates: While not as intense as some of the other exercises on this list, yoga, and Pilates can help improve flexibility, balance, and core strength, which can be beneficial for weight loss.

Remember, while exercise is important for weight loss, it's also essential to maintain a healthy diet and lifes.

C.How much exercise is needed for weight loss

The amount of exercise needed for weight loss depends on several factors, including your current weight, body composition, exercise habits, and overall health. In general, a combination of regular exercise and a healthy diet is necessary for effective weight loss.
The American College of Sports Medicine (ACSM) recommends at least 150 minutes of moderate-intensity exercise or 75 minutes of vigorous-intensity exercise per week to promote weight loss. This can be achieved through a variety of activities, such as brisk walking, running, cycling, swimming, or strength training. However, it's important to note that the amount of exercise needed for weight loss can vary widely from person to person, and may also depend on factors such as genetics, hormones, and stress levels. Additionally,

exercise alone may not be sufficient for weight loss if dietary changes are not also made.

Therefore, it's recommended to consult with a healthcare professional or a certified personal trainer to develop a personalized exercise plan that takes into account your individual needs and goals.

Chapter 4

Lifestyle changes

A.Importance of lifestyle changes on weight loss

A.Importance of lifestyle changes on weight loss Lifestyle changes can have a significant impact on weight loss. Making changes to your diet, exercise routine, and overall habits can help you lose weight and maintain a healthy weight in the long term.

Here are some of the ways lifestyle changes can contribute to weight loss:

1. Caloric intake: The most effective way to lose weight is to create a calorie deficit, which means burning more calories than you consume. Eating a healthy, balanced diet that includes plenty of fruits, vegetables, whole grains, lean proteins, and healthy fats can help you reduce your calorie intake and lose weight.

2. Exercise: Regular physical activity is essential for weight loss. Exercise burns calories boost metabolism, and builds muscle, which can help you burn more calories even when you're not exercising. Strive to engage in at least 150 minutes of moderate-intensity physical activity per week, such as brisk walking, cycling, or swimming.

3. Rest: Getting enough rest is crucial for weight loss. Lack of rest can disrupt hormones that regulate hunger and appetite, leading to overeating and weight gain. Strive to also engage in 7-9 hours of sleep per night.

4. Stress management: Stress can lead to overeating and weight gain. Finding healthy ways to manage stress, such as

meditation, yoga, or deep breathing, can help you stay on track with your weight loss goals.

5. Habits: Changing unhealthy habits, such as drinking sugary beverages or snacking late at night, can make a big difference in weight loss. Replace these habits with healthier alternatives, such as drinking water or herbal tea and snacking on fruits and vegetables.

Overall, making sustainable lifestyle changes can help you achieve and maintain a healthy weight, improve your overall health, and reduce your risk of chronic diseases.

B.Sleep and its role in weight loss

Obtaining sufficient sleep is a fundamental aspect of maintaining a healthy weight. Research has shown that sleep plays a critical role in regulating hormones that control appetite and metabolism.

When sleep is inadequate, the body increases the production of ghrelin, a hormone that triggers appetite, and reduces the production of leptin, a hormone that suppresses appetite. This can lead to overeating and weight gain.

Sleep deprivation can also affect your metabolism. When you're tired, your body burns fewer calories at rest than it would if you were well-rested. This means that even if you're eating the same number of calories as you normally would, you may still gain weight if you're not getting enough sleep.

Additionally, lack of sleep can lead to increased levels of the stress hormone cortisol, which can trigger your body to store fat, especially in the abdominal area. Overall, getting enough sleep is an important part of a healthy lifestyle, and can help support weight loss efforts. According to the National Sleep Foundation, it is recommended that adults strive to get 7-9 hours of sleep per night.

C.Stress and its impact on weight loss:

Stress can have a significant impact on weight loss efforts. When you experience stress, your body releases cortisol, which is a hormone that can increase your appetite and make you crave unhealthy foods. In addition, cortisol can cause your body to store fat, particularly in the abdominal area.

Here are some ways that stress can impact weight loss:

1. Increased appetite: When you're stressed, your body produces more cortisol, which can increase your appetite and make you crave high-calorie foods.

2. Emotional eating: Stress can also trigger emotional eating, which is when you turn to food to cope with stress, anxiety, or other negative emotions.

3. Decreased motivation: Stress can make it harder to stick to healthy habits, such as exercising regularly and eating a balanced diet. This can lead to a decrease in motivation to maintain a weight loss plan.

4. Sleep disturbances: Chronic stress can disrupt your sleep, which can negatively impact your weight loss efforts. Sleep deprivation can increase your appetite and interfere with your

body's ability to regulate hormones that control hunger.

5. Hormonal changes: Stress can alter the levels of various hormones in your body, including cortisol, insulin, and thyroid hormones. These hormonal changes can impact your metabolism and make it harder to lose weight.

D.Other lifestyle changes for weight loss

Weight loss can be achieved through a variety of lifestyle changes in addition to a healthy diet and regular exercise. Here are some additional lifestyle changes that may help with weight loss:

1. Get Enough Sleep: Lack of sleep can cause weight gain by disrupting hormones that regulate appetite and metabolism. Strive to achieve 7-9 hours of sleep per night.

2. Minimize Stress: Persistent stress can result in overeating and weight gain. Discover approaches to manage and mitigate stress, such as practicing meditation or yoga, or seeking counsel from a therapist.

3. Stay Hydrated: Adequate water intake can induce feelings of fullness and diminish appetite. Strive to consume a minimum of eight 8-ounce glasses of water each day.

4. Avoid Sugary Drinks: Sugary drinks like soda and juice can add a lot of calories to your diet without providing much nutrition. Stick to water, unsweetened tea, or black coffee instead.

5. Eat Mindfully: Pay attention to your food while you eat, and avoid distractions like television or smartphones. Eating mindfully can help you eat less and enjoy your food more.

6. Practice Portion Control: Use smaller plates and bowls, and measure your food to avoid overeating.

7. Get Active Throughout the Day: Find ways to be active throughout the day, such as taking the stairs instead of the elevator, or going for a walk during your lunch break.

8. Surround Yourself with Support: Surround yourself with people who will encourage and support your weight loss efforts.

Join a weight loss support group or enlist the help of a friend or family member.

Remember that making lifestyle changes for weight loss takes time and effort, but the benefits are well worth it.

Chapter 5

Weight loss strategies

A.Fad diets and their limitations

Fad diets are diets that are popular for a short period of time, often promoted by celebrities, social media influencers, or authors of popular diet books. These diets usually promise quick weight loss, improved health, or both, but they are often not backed by scientific evidence and may have limitations. Here are some limitations of fad diets:

1. Unsustainable: Many fad diets are difficult to sustain over the long term because they often require drastic changes in eating habits or eliminate entire food

groups. This can lead to feelings of deprivation, making it difficult to stick to the diet for the long term.

2. Nutrient deficiencies: Some fad diets eliminate entire food groups or restrict calories to such a degree that nutrient deficiencies can occur. This can lead to health problems such as fatigue, weakness, and immune system dysfunction.

3. Lack of scientific evidence: Many fad diets are not based on scientific evidence and are often promoted by people who are not qualified to give dietary advice. This can lead to confusion and misinformation about what constitutes a healthy diet.

4. Yo-yo dieting: Fad diets often promote rapid weight loss, but this weight loss is often not sustainable. When people go off the diet, they often regain the weight they lost, leading to a cycle of yo-yo dieting that can be harmful to their health.

5. Risk of eating disorders: Some fad diets can promote unhealthy eating habits that can lead to eating disorders such as anorexia or bulimia.

5. Lack of individualization: Fad diets are often a one-size-fits-all approach that does not take into account an individual's unique dietary needs or medical history.
6. May not promote long-term health: Many fad diets focus on short-term weight loss goals rather than promoting long-term health. This could result in future health complications. It's important to remember that a healthy diet should be balanced and sustainable and that individual dietary needs may vary. Seek advice from a certified healthcare practitioner prior to commencing any diet or fitness regiment.

B.Healthy and efficient weight reduction techniques:

Losing weight can be challenging, but there are safe and effective strategies that can help you reach your goals. Here are some tips:
1. Establish a negative energy balance: To achieve weight loss, you must expend more energy than you consume. This can be attained by adopting a nourishing and balanced diet consisting of

ample fruits, vegetables, whole grains, lean protein, and beneficial fats.

2. Engage in consistent physical activity: Consistent exercise can enhance caloric expenditure and boost metabolic rate. Strive for a minimum of 150 minutes of moderate-intensity cardiorespiratory exercise or 75 minutes of vigorous-intensity cardiorespiratory exercise per week.

3. Keep track of your food intake: Keeping a food diary or using a mobile app to track your food intake can help you monitor your calorie intake and make better food choices.

4. Obtain sufficient rest: Inadequate sleep can result in weight gain by disturbing hormones that control hunger and metabolism. Strive for a minimum of 7-8 hours of sleep per night.

5. Consume abundant water: Hydrating with water can induce satiety and lower calorie consumption. Strive for a minimum of 8 glasses of water per day.

6. Avoid sugary and processed foods: Sugary and processed foods can be high in calories and low in nutrients. Choose whole, nutrient-dense foods instead.

7. Consider weight loss medication or surgery: If you have a BMI of 30 or higher or a BMI of 27 or higher with weight-related health problems, weight loss medication or surgery may be an option to help you reach your goals. However, these options should only be considered after consulting with a healthcare provider.

Remember, sustainable weight loss takes time and requires lifestyle changes. Be patient and consistent, and seek support from friends, family, or a healthcare professional if needed.

C.Choosing weight loss plan that works for you

Choosing a weight loss plan that works for you can be a challenging process, but with careful consideration and planning, you can find the right approach for your needs and goals. Here are some steps to help you choose a weight loss plan that works for you:

1. Determine your goals: Before you start looking for a weight loss plan, you should determine your weight loss goals. Do you want to lose a specific amount of weight or do you want to adopt a healthier lifestyle? Knowing your goals will help you choose a plan that is tailored to your needs.

2. Consult a healthcare professional: Before embarking on any weight loss plan, it is essential to consult with a healthcare professional to ensure that it is safe and appropriate for you. They can also help you determine the best approach based on your medical history, medications, and any other health concerns.

3. Consider your lifestyle: When choosing a weight loss plan, consider your lifestyle and how it will fit into your daily routine. If you have a busy schedule, you may want to consider a plan that doesn't require a lot of meal prep or gym time.

4. Research different plans: There are many weight loss plans available, from low-carb diets to

meal replacement programs. Research different plans and consider the pros and cons of each approach. Look for plans that have been scientifically proven to work and have long-term success rates.

5. Choose a plan that you can stick to: The key to successful weight loss is finding a plan that you can stick to in the long term. Choose a plan that you enjoy and that fits your personality and preferences. If you don't like the foods or exercises in a plan, you won't be able to stick to it.

Pricing page

6. Track your progress:
Once you have chosen a weight loss plan, track your progress and make adaptations as demanded. Keep a food journal and track your exercises to cover your progress and stay motivated. Remember, there's no one - size-fits- all approach to weight loss. Choose a plan that works for you and do not be hysterical to make adaptations along the way. With the right approach, you can achieve your weight loss pretensions and borrow a healthier lifestyle.

D.Tips for successful weight loss

Set realistic pretensions rather than aiming for an unrealistic weight loss target, set attainable pretensions that are specific, measurable, and time-bound. This will help you stay motivated and focused. Keep a food journal Write down what you eat and drink every day. This will help you keep track of your calorie input and identify any unhealthy eating patterns that you need to change. Eat a healthy, balanced diet Focus on eating nutrients I.e foods similar to fruits, vegetables, whole grains, spare tissue builders, and healthy fats. Avoid reused foods, sticky drinks, and high-calorie snacks. Exercise regularly Aim for at least 30 twinkles of moderate-intensity exercise most days of the week. You can choose the conditioning that you enjoy, similar to walking, jogging, swimming, or cycling.
Lack of sleep can get into a challenge in your metabolism and increase your craving for food. Aim for 7- 8 hours of sleep

each night to help support your weight loss goals. Stay doused Drinking enough water can help you feel full and reduce your appetite. Strive for at least 8- 10 servings of water per day.

Find a support system compassing yourself with people who'll encourage and motivate you to reach your weight loss pretensions. This can be a family, musketeers, or a support group. Case Losing weight takes time, and it's important to be patient and patient. Do not get discouraged if you do not see results incontinently. Keep making healthy choices, and weight loss will follow.

Chapter 6

Weight maintenance

A.The importance of weight maintenance

Weight maintenance is essential for good health and well-being. It refers to the ability to maintain a stable weight, neither gaining nor losing weight excessively. The importance of weight maintenance includes:

1. Healthy Body Weight: Maintaining a healthy weight can reduce the risk of many health problems, such as heart disease, diabetes, high blood pressure, stroke, and certain types of cancer.

2. Improved Energy Levels: Maintaining a stable weight can help improve energy levels and prevent fatigue.

3. Mental Health: Being at a healthy weight can also improve mental health and well-being. Excessive weight gain or loss can lead to depression, anxiety, and other mental health issues.

4. Better Sleep: Maintaining a healthy weight can also improve sleep quality and reduce the risk of sleep apnea.

5. Improved Mobility: Being at a healthy weight can improve mobility, making it easier to move around and perform everyday tasks.

6. Reduced Healthcare Costs: Maintaining a healthy weight can also reduce healthcare costs associated with obesity-related health problems.

Overall, weight maintenance is crucial for good health and can improve the quality of life in many ways. It's important to adopt healthy habits, such as a balanced diet and regular exercise, to maintain a healthy weight.

B.Strategies for maintaining weight

Maintaining a healthy weight can be challenging, but there are several strategies you can follow to make it easier:

1. Follow a balanced diet: Eat a diet rich in fruits, vegetables, lean protein, and whole grains. Avoid processed foods and excessive amounts of sugar, salt, and unhealthy fats.

2. Practice portion control: Be mindful of how much you eat and use smaller plates and bowls to help control portion sizes.

3. Stay hydrated: Drink plenty of water throughout the day to keep your body hydrated and to help you feel full.

4. Incorporate physical activity into your daily routine: Aim for at least 30 minutes of moderate-intensity exercise most days of

the week, such as brisk walking, cycling, or swimming.

5. Obtain sufficient sleep: Insufficient sleep can disturb the hormones responsible for controlling appetite and metabolism, rendering it more difficult to sustain a healthy weight.

6. Monitor your weight regularly: Weigh yourself weekly or monthly to track your progress and catch any changes early.

7. Seek support: Consider joining a weight loss support group or enlisting the help of a registered dietitian or personal trainer to help you stay on track.

Remember that maintaining a healthy weight is not just about diet and exercise but also about making sustainable lifestyle changes that you can stick to over the long term.

C.Coping with weight regain

Weight regain can be a frustrating experience, but it's important to remember that it's a normal part of the weight loss journey. Here are some tips for coping with weight regain:

1. Practice self-compassion: Avoid being harsh on yourself for regaining weight. Acknowledge that weight loss is a process with its own share of setbacks and difficulties. Be kind to yourself and remind yourself that you're making a sincere effort.

2. Reassess your goals: Take some time to reassess your weight loss goals. Are they realistic and achievable? If not, adjust them so that they are more attainable. Keep in mind that gradual and consistent weight loss is more viable in the long term.

3. Focus on healthy habits: Instead of focusing solely on the number on the scale, shift your focus to developing healthy habits that will help you maintain a healthy weight over time. This might include making healthier food choices, getting regular exercise, and practicing stress management techniques.

4. Seek support: Surround yourself with a supportive community, whether it's friends and family, a weight loss support group, or a healthcare

professional. Having a network of supporters can aid in keeping you motivated and focused on your goals.

5. Persist: Lastly, keep pushing forward and don't give up. Remember that weight loss is a journey with ups and downs, and setbacks are a normal part of the process. Keep working towards your goals and celebrate your successes along the way.

Conclusion

A.Summary of essential factors for revealing the mysteries of weight loss

1. Energy deficit: This refers to the situation where your body is burning more energy than it is taking in through food and drink, leading to weight loss. Other possible terms that could be used include "negative energy balance" or "energy shortfall.

2. Balanced diet: A balanced diet that includes a variety of fruits, vegetables, whole grains, lean proteins, and healthy fats is

crucial for weight loss. Avoid processed and high-calorie foods.

3. Mindful eating: Be mindful of the amount of food you consume by paying attention to your hunger cues and eating slowly. Use smaller meal dishes and utensils to assist you with portion control.

4. Hydration: Drinking enough water is essential for weight loss. It helps flush toxins out of your body and can curb your appetite.

5. Exercise: Regular exercise can help you burn calories and build muscle, which boosts your metabolism. Strive to accumulate a minimum of 150 minutes of moderate-intensity exercise each week.

6. Rest: Sufficient rest is crucial for achieving weight loss goals. Lack of adequate rest can disrupt your hormones and make it harder to lose weight.

7. Stress management: High levels of stress can cause weight gain. Discover strategies to cope with stress, such as practicing meditation, engaging in yoga, or utilizing deep breathing exercises."

8. Regularity: Regularity is critical for achieving and maintaining weight loss. Stick to your plan, and don't give up if you have setbacks.

9. Accountability: Having someone to hold you accountable can help you stay on track with your weight loss goals. Explore the possibility of joining a support group, or enlisting the assistance of a personal trainer or nutritionist.

10. Patience: Weight loss is a gradual process, and it takes time to see results. Be patient and don't get discouraged if you don't see immediate changes.

B.Encouragement for Weight Loss

Congratulations on making the decision to take action toward achieving a healthy weight! Here are some words of encouragement to help you on your journey:

1. Start small: Don't try to make all the changes just at once. Emphasize implementing small, achievable modifications to your dietary and exercise habits that

you can maintain over time. This could include swapping out sugary drinks for water, taking the stairs instead of the elevator, or going for a walk after dinner.

2. Set realistic goals: Losing weight is a journey, not a sprint. Set realistic goals for yourself that are achievable within a reasonable timeframe. Recognize and acknowledge your accomplishments throughout your journey, no matter how minor they may seem

3. Build a support system: Surround yourself with people who will encourage and support you on your journey. This could be a friend or family member, a support group, or a health coach.

4. Be patient: Weight loss takes time, and it's important to be patient with yourself. Stay encouraged and persistent, even if you do not observe immediate changes in your progress. Focus on the progress you are making, and keep moving forward.

5. Stay positive: A positive attitude can make all the difference in achieving your goals. Focus on the benefits of living a healthy lifestyle, and

remind yourself of why you started on this journey in the first place.

Remember, taking action towards a healthy weight is one of the most important things you can do for your overall health and well-being. Stay determined, stay dedicated, and you will achieve your goals!

www.ingramcontent.com/pod-product-compliance
Lightning Source LLC
Chambersburg PA
CBHW071113220526
45467CB00004B/1858